Anti-Inflammatory Side Dish Book

Easy and tasy recipes to Help Your Immune System and stay fit

Natalie Worley

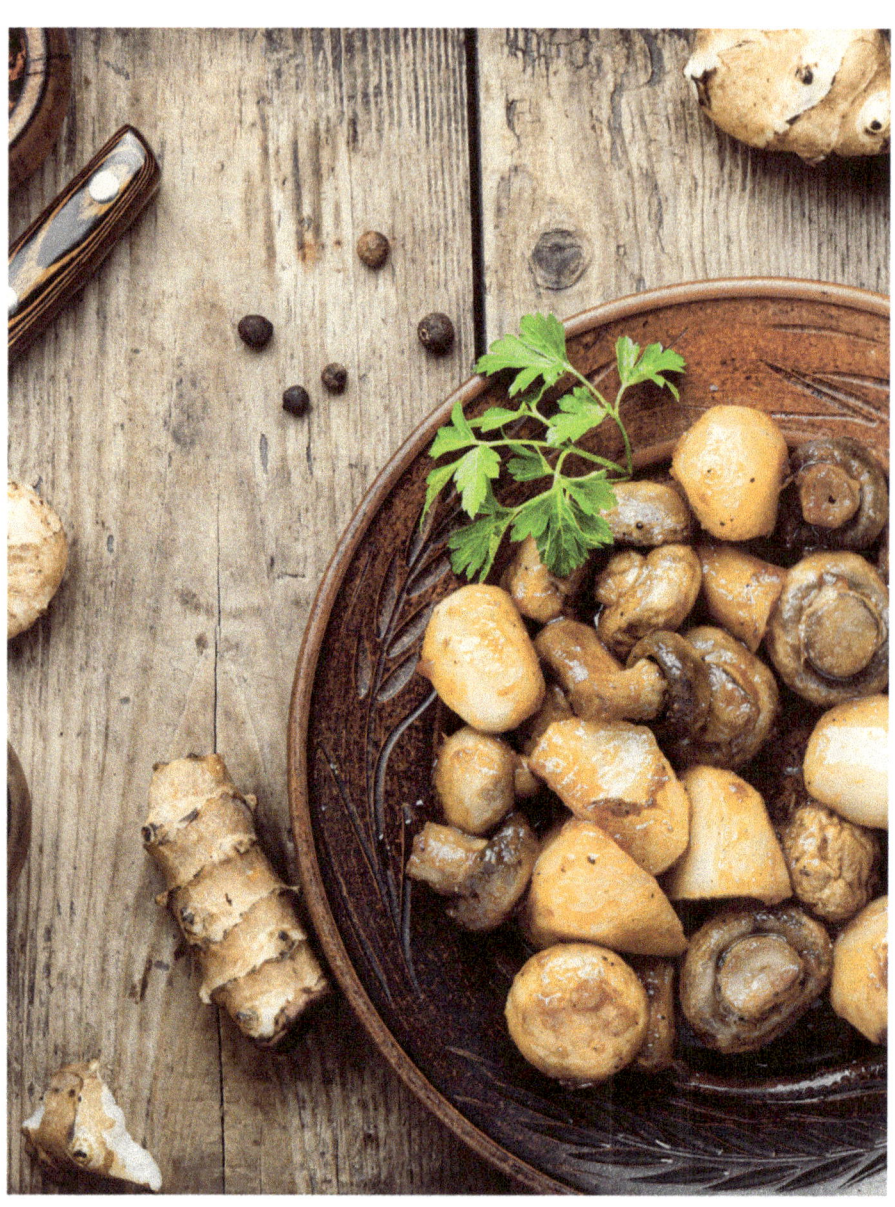

© copyright 2021 – all rights reserved.

the content contained within this book may not be reproduced, duplicated or transmitted without direct written permission from the author or the publisher.

under no circumstances will any blame or legal responsibility be held against the publisher, or author, for any damages, reparation, or monetary loss due to the information contained within this book. either directly or indirectly.

legal notice:

this book is copyright protected. this book is only for personal use. you cannot amend, distribute, sell, use, quote or paraphrase any part, or the content within this book, without the consent of the author or publisher.

disclaimer notice:

please note the information contained within this document is for educational and entertainment purposes only. all effort has been executed to present accurate, up to date, and reliable, complete information. no warranties of any kind are declared or implied. readers acknowledge that the author is not engaging in the rendering of legal, financial, medical or professional advice. the content within this book has been derived from various sources. please consult a licensed professional before attempting any techniques outlined in this book.

by reading this document, the reader agrees that under no circumstances is the author responsible for any losses, direct or indirect, which are incurred as a result of the use of information contained within this document, including, but not limited to, — errors, omissions, or inaccuracies.

Table of Contents

Garden Vegetable Mash 6
Spicy and Cheesy Roasted Artichokes 9
Cheesy Stuffed Peppers with Cauliflower Rice 11
Broccoli and Bacon Soup 13
Aromatic Kale with Garlic 15
Spanish-Style Keto Slaw 17
Cheesy Breakfast Broccoli Casserole 19
Cauli Mac and Cheese 21
Baked Vegetable Side 24
Shrimp Fra Diavolo 25
Zucchini and Cheese Gratin 27
Soy Garlic Mushrooms 29
Old Bay Chicken Wings 31
Tofu Stuffed Peppers 34
Air Fryer Garlic Chicken Wings 36
Sautéed Brussels Sprouts 38
Bacon Jalapeno Poppers 39
Basil Keto Crackers 41
Crispy Keto Pork Bites 43
Fat Burger Bombs 45
Onion Cheese Muffins 47
Bacon-Flavored Kale Chips 50
Keto-Approved Trail Mix 52
Reese Cups 53
Curry 'n Poppy Devilled Eggs 55

- Bacon and Cheddar Cheese Balls ... 58
- Cheese Roll-Ups the Keto Way ... 60
- Cheddar Cheese Chips ... 61
- Cardamom and Cinnamon Fat Bombs ... 62
- No Cook Coconut and Chocolate Bars ... 64
- Coleslaw ... 66
- Roasted Zucchini and Pumpkin Cubes ... 67
- Chile Casserole ... 69
- Pickled Jalapeno ... 71
- Naan ... 73
- Sauteed Tomato Cabbage ... 76
- Tender Radicchio ... 78
- Green Salad with Walnuts ... 80
- Jicama Slaw ... 82
- Peanut Slaw ... 84
- White Mushroom Saute ... 86
- Caesar Salad ... 89
- Cranberry Relish ... 91
- Vegetable Tots ... 93
- Hasselback Zucchini ... 95
- Lime Fennel Bulb ... 97
- Baked Garlic ... 99
- Roasted Okra ... 101
- Broccoli Gratin ... 103
- Cayenne Pepper Green Beans ... 106

Garden Vegetable Mash

Prep Time: 15 minutes | **Serve:** 3

- 1 ½ tablespoons butter
- 4 tablespoons cream cheese
- ½ pound cauliflower florets
- ½ pound broccoli florets
- 1/2 teaspoon garlic powder

1.Parboil the broccoli and cauliflower for about 10 minutes until they have softened. Mash them with a potato masher.

2.Add in garlic powder, cream cheese, and butter; mix to combine well. Season with salt and black pepper to taste.

Nutrition: 162 Calories; 12.8g Fat; 7.2g Carbs; 4.7g Protein; 3.5g Fiber

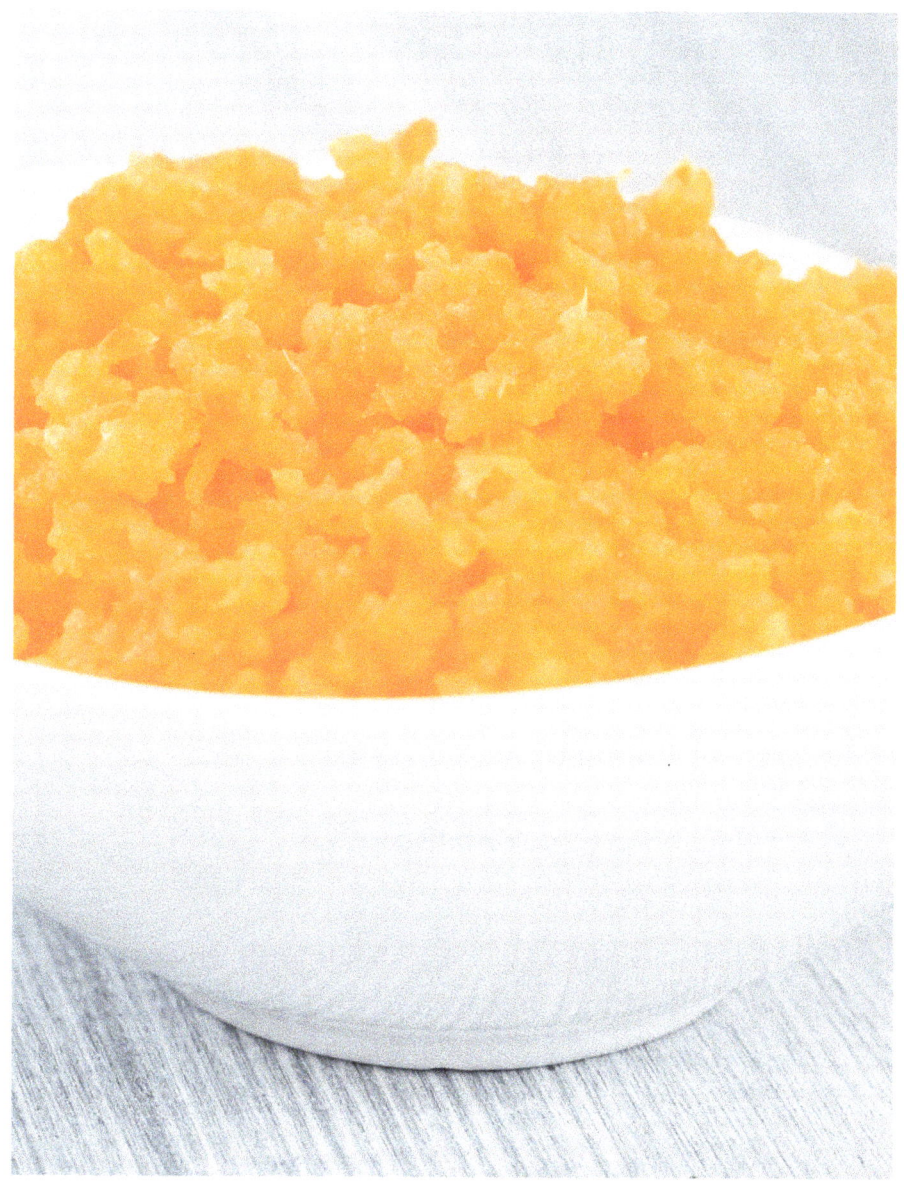

Spicy and Cheesy Roasted Artichokes

Prep Time: 1 hour 10 minutes | **Serve:** 2

- 2 small-sized globe artichokes, cut off the stalks
- 2 tablespoons butter, melted
- 2 tablespoons fresh lime juice
- 1/2 cup Romano cheese, grated
- 2 tablespoons mayonnaise

1.Start by preheating your oven to 420 degrees F.

2.To prepare your artichokes, discard the tough outer layers; cut off about 3/4 inches from the top. Slice them in half lengthwise.

3. Toss your artichokes with butter and fresh lime juice; season with the salt and pepper to taste.

4. Top with the grated Romano cheese; wrap your artichokes in foil and roast them in the preheated oven for about 1 hour.

Nutrition: 368 Calories; 33g Fat; 7.2g Carbs; 10.6g Protein; 3.8g Fiber

Cheesy Stuffed Peppers with Cauliflower Rice

Prep Time: 45 minutes | **Serve:** 6

- 6 medium-sized bell peppers, deveined and cleaned
- 1 cup cauliflower rice
- 1/2 cup tomato sauce with garlic and onion
- 1 pound ground turkey
- 1/2 cup Cheddar cheese, shredded

1.Heat 2 tablespoons of olive oil in a frying pan over medium-high heat. Then, cook ground turkey until nicely browned or about 5 minutes.

2.Add in cauliflower rice and season with salt and black pepper. Continue to cook for 3 to 4 minutes more.

3.Add in tomato sauce. Stuff the peppers with this filling and cover with a piece of aluminum foil.

4.Bake in the preheated oven at 390 degrees F for 17 to 20 minutes. Remove the foil, top with cheese, and bake for a further 10 to 13 minutes. Bon appétit!

Nutrition: 244 Calories; 12.9g Fat; 3.2g Carbs; 1g Fiber; 16.5g Protein;

Broccoli and Bacon Soup

Prep Time: 20 minutes | **Serve:** 4

- 1 head broccoli, broken into small florets
- 1 carrot, chopped
- 1 celery, chopped
- 1/2 cup full-fat yogurt
- 2 slices bacon, chopped

1. Fry the bacon in a soup pot over a moderate flame; reserve.

2. Then, cook the carrots, celery and broccoli in the bacon fat. Season with salt and pepper to taste.

3. Pour in 4 cups of water or vegetable stock, bringing to a boil. Turn the temperature to a simmer and continue to cook, partially covered, for 10 to 15 minutes longer.

4.Add in yogurt and remove from heat. Puree your soup with an immersion blender until your desired consistency is reached.

5.Garnish with the reserved bacon and serve.

Nutrition: 95 Calories; 7.6g Fat; 4.1g Carbs; 3g Protein; 1g Fiber

Aromatic Kale with Garlic

Prep Time: 20 minutes | **Serve:** 3

- 1/2 tablespoon olive oil
- 1/2 cup cottage cheese, creamed
- 1/2 teaspoon sea salt
- 1 teaspoon fresh garlic, chopped
- 9 ounces kale, torn into pieces

1. Heat the olive oil in a pot over medium-high flame. Once hot, fry the garlic until just tender and fragrant or about 30 seconds.

2. Add in kale and continue to cook for 8 to 10 minutes until all liquid evaporates.

3. Add in cottage cheese and sea salt, remove from heat, and stir until everything is combined. Bon appétit!

Nutrition: 93 Calories; 4.4g Fat; 6.1g Carbs; 7.1g Protein; 2.7g Fiber

Spanish-Style Keto Slaw

Prep Time: 10 minutes | **Serve:** 4

- 1 teaspoon fresh garlic, minced
- 4 tablespoons tahini (sesame paste
- ½ pound Napa cabbage, shredded
- 2 cups arugula, torn into pieces
- 1 Spanish onion, thinly sliced into rings

1. Make a dressing by whisking the garlic and tahini; add in 2 teaspoons of balsamic vinegar along with salt and black pepper.
2. In a salad bowl, combine Napa cabbage, arugula, and Spanish onion. Toss the salad with dressing.
3. Garnish with sesame seeds if desired and serve.

Nutrition: 122 Calories; 9.1g Fat; 5.9g Carbs; 4.5g Protein; 3g Fiber

Cheesy Breakfast Broccoli Casserole

Prep Time: 40 minutes | **Serve:** 4

- 1 (1/2-poundhead broccoli, broken into florets
- 1 cup cooked ham, chopped
- 1/2 cup Greek-style yogurt
- 1 cup Mexican cheese, shredded
- 1/2 teaspoon butter, melted

1.Begin by preheating an oven to 350 degrees F. Now, butter the bottom and sides of a casserole dish with melted butter.

2.Cook broccoli for 6 to 7 minutes until it is "mashable". Mash the broccoli with a potato masher.

3.Now, stir in Greek-style yogurt, Mexican cheese, and cooked ham. Season with Mexican spice blend, if desired.

4.Press the cheese/broccoli mixture in the buttered casserole dish. Bake in the preheated oven for 20 to 23 minutes.

Nutrition: 188 Calories; 11.3g Fat; 5.7g Carbs; 14.9g Protein; 1.1g Fiber

Cauli Mac and Cheese

Prep Time: 15 Min | **Cook Time:** 15 Min | **Serve:** 6

- 1 head cauliflower, blanched and cut into florets
- ½ cup nutritional yeast
- 1 cup heavy cream
- 5 tablespoons butter, melted
- 1 ½ cup cheddar cheese Salt and pepper to taste
- ½ cup water or milk

1. In a heat-proof dish, place the cauliflower florets. Set aside. In a mixing bowl, combine the rest of the ingredients. Pour over the cauliflower florets.
2. Bake in a 350OF preheated oven for 15 minutes. Place in containers and put the proper label. Store in the fridge

and consume before 3 days. Microwave or bake in the oven first before eating.

Nutrition: Calories: 329; Fat: 30.3g; Carbs: 10.1g; Protein: 12.1g

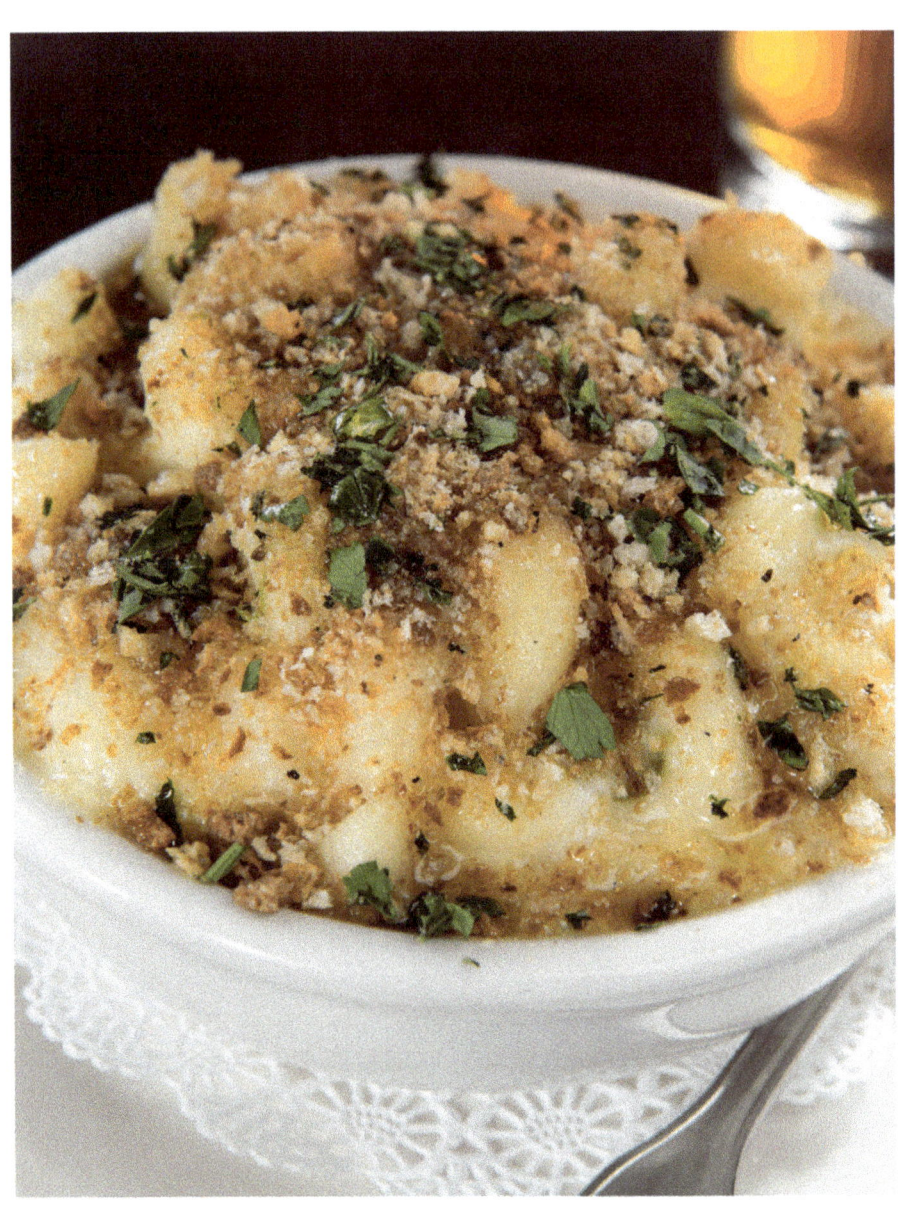

Baked Vegetable Side

Prep Time: Min | **Cook Time:** 15 Min | **Serve:** 4

- 2 large zucchinis, sliced
- 2 bell peppers, sliced
- ½ cup peeled garlic cloves, sliced A dash of oregano
- 4 tablespoons olive oil Salt and pepper to taste

1. Place all ingredients in a mixing bowl. Stir to coat everything. Place in a baking sheet.
2. Bake in a 350ºF preheated oven for 15 minutes.

Nutrition: Calories: 191; Fat: 23.0g; Carbs: 12.0g; Protein: 3.0g

Shrimp Fra Diavola

Prep Time: 15 Min | **Cook Time:** 5 Min | **Serve:** 3

- 3 tablespoons butter
- 1 onion, diced
- 5 cloves of garlic, minced
- 1 teaspoon red pepper flakes
- ¼ pound shrimps, shelled
- 2 tablespoons olive oil Salt and pepper to taste

1. Heat the butter and the olive oil in a skillet and sauté the onion and garlic until fragrant.

2. Stir in the red pepper flakes and shrimps. Season with salt and pepper to taste.

3. Stir for 3 minutes.

Nutrition: Calories: 145; Fat: 32.1g; Carbs: 4.5g;

Protein: 21.0g

Zucchini and Cheese Gratin

Prep Time: 15 Min | **Cook Time:** 15 Min | **Serve:** 8

- 5 tablespoons butter
- 1 onion, sliced
- ½ cup heavy cream
- 4 cups raw zucchini, sliced
- 1 ½ cups shredded pepper Jack cheese Salt and pepper to taste

1. Place all ingredients in a mixing bowl and give a good stir to incorporate everything.

2. Pour the mixture in a heat-proof baking dish.

3. Place in a 350°F preheated oven and bake for 15 minutes.

Nutrition: Calories: 280; Fat: 20.0g; Carbs: 5.0g; Protein: 8.0g

Soy Garlic Mushrooms

Prep Time: 20 Min | **Cook Time:** 10 Min | **Serve:** 8

- 2 pounds mushrooms, sliced
- 3 tablespoons olive oil
- 2 cloves of garlic, minced
- ¼ ncup coconut aminos Salt and pepper to taste

1. Place all ingredients in a dish and mix until well-combined. Allow to marinate for 2 hours in the fridge.
2. In a large saucepan on medium fire, add mushrooms and sauté for 8 minutes.
3. Season with pepper and salt to taste.

Nutrition: Calories: 383; Fat: 10.9g; Carbs: 86.0g; Protein: 6.2g

Old Bay Chicken Wings

Prep Time: 5 Min | **Cook Time:** 30 Min | **Serve:** 4

- 3 pounds chicken wings
- ¾ cup almond flour
- 1 tablespoon old bay spices
- 1 teaspoon lemon juice, freshly squeezed ½ cup butter
- Salt and pepper to taste

1. Preheat oven to 400oF.
2. In a mixing bowl, combine all ingredients except for the butter.
3. Place in an even layer in a baking sheet.
4. Bake for 30 minutes. Halfway through the cooking time, shake the fryer basket for even cooking.

5.Once cooked, drizzle with melted butter.

Nutrition: Calories: 640; Fat: 59.2g; Carbs: 1.6g; Protein: 52.5g

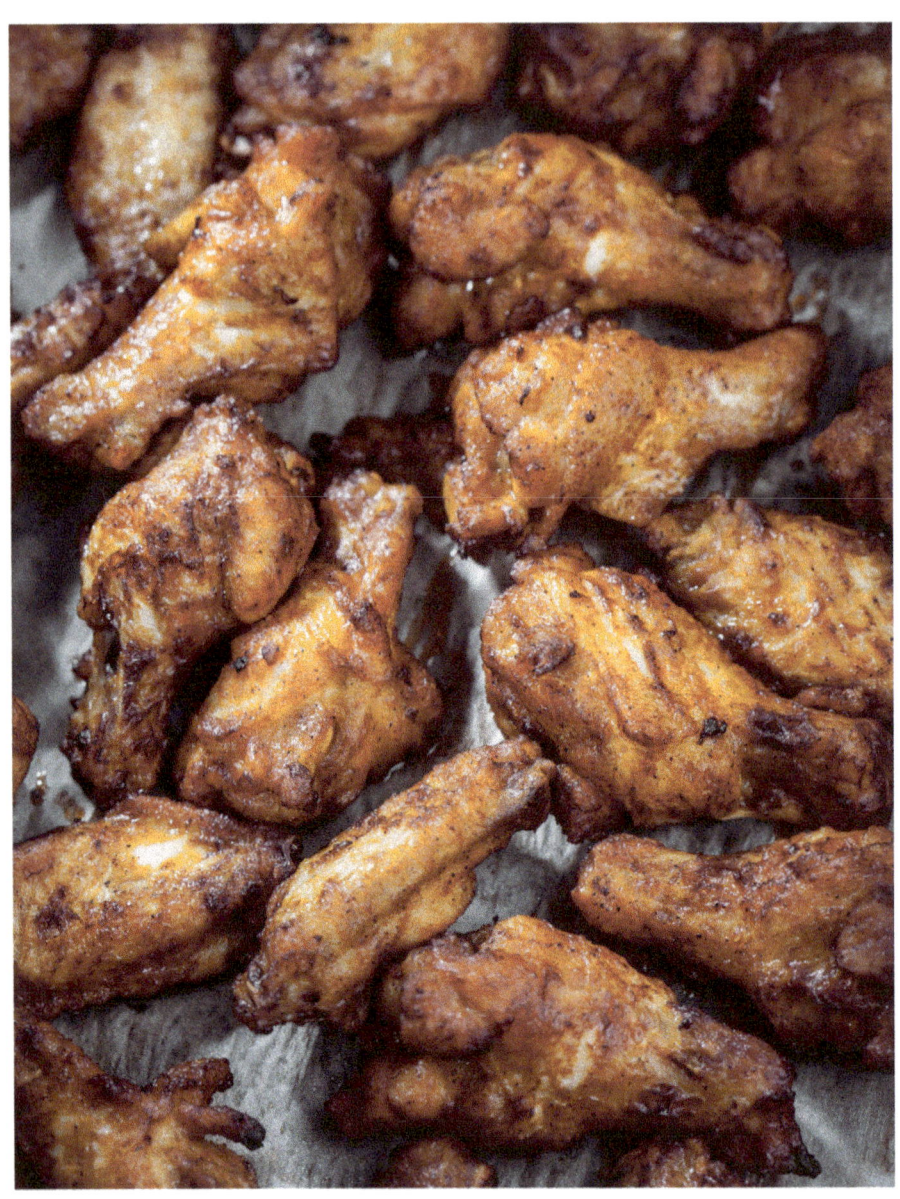

Tofu Stuffed Peppers

Prep Time: 5 Min | **Cook Time:** 10 Min | **Serve:** 8

- 1 package firm tofu, crumbled
- 1 onion, finely chopped
- ½ teaspoon turmeric powder
- 1 teaspoon coriander powder
- 8 banana peppers, top end sliced and seeded Salt and pepper to taste
- 3 tablespoons oil

1.Preheat oven to 400oF.

2.In a mixing bowl, combine the tofu, onion, coconut oil, turmeric powder, red chili powder, coriander power, and salt. Mix until well-combined.

3.Scoop the tofu mixture into the hollows of the banana peppers.

4.Place the stuffed peppers in one layer in a lightly greased baking sheet.

5.Cook for 10 minutes.

Nutrition: Calories: 67; Fat: 5.6g; Carbs: 4.1g; Protein: 1.2g

Air Fryer Garlic Chicken Wings

Prep Time: 5 Min | **Cook Time:** 25 Min | **Serve:** 4

- 16 pieces chicken wings
- ¾ cup almond flour
- 4 tablespoons minced garlic
- ¼ cup butter, melted Salt and pepper to taste
- 2 tablespoons stevia powder

1. Preheat oven to 400oF.

2. In a mixing bowl, combine the chicken wings, almond flour, stevia powder, and garlic Season with salt and pepper to taste.

3. Place in a lightly greased cookie sheet in an even layer and cook for 25 minutes.

4. Halfway through the cooking time, turnover chicken.

5.Once cooked, place in a bowl and drizzle with melted butter. Toss to coat.

Nutrition: Calories: 365; Fat: 26.9g; Carbs: 7.8g; Protein: 23.7g

Sautéed Brussels Sprouts

Prep Time: 5 Min | **Cook Time:** 8 Min | **Serve:** 4

- 2 cups Brussels sprouts, halved
- 1 tablespoon balsamic vinegar
- Salt and pepper to taste
- 2 tablespoons olive oil

1. Place a saucepan on medium high fire and heat oil for a minute.
2. Add all ingredients and sauté for 7 minutes.
3. Season with pepper and salt.

Nutrition: Calories: 82; Fat: 6.8g; Carbs: 4.6g; Protein: 1.5g

Bacon Jalapeno Poppers

Prep Time: 15 Min | **Cook Time:** 10 Min | **Serve:** 8

- 4-ounce cream cheese
- ¼ cup cheddar cheese, shredded
- 1 teaspoon paprika
- 16 fresh jalapenos, sliced lengthwise and seeded
- 16 strips of uncured bacon, cut into half Salt and pepper to taste

1. Preheat oven to 400oF.

2. In a mixing bowl, mix the cream cheese, cheddar cheese, salt, and paprika until well-combined.

3. Scoop half a teaspoon onto each half of jalapeno peppers.

4.Use a thin strip of bacon and wrap it around the cheese-filled jalapeno half.

5.Place in a single layer in a lightly greased baking sheet and roast for 10 minutes.

Nutrition: Calories: 225; Fat: 18.9g; Carbs: 3.2g; Protein: 10.6g

Basil Keto Crackers

Prep Time: 30 Min | **Cook Time:** 15 Min | **Serve:** 6

- 1 ¼ cups almond flour
- ½ teaspoon baking powder ¼ teaspoon dried basil powder
- A pinch of cayenne pepper powder 1 clove of garlic, minced
- Salt and pepper to taste 3 tablespoons oil

1. Preheat oven to 350oF and lightly grease a cookie sheet with cooking spray. Mix everything in a mixing bowl to create a dough.
2. Transfer the dough on a clean and flat working surface and spread out until 2mm thick. Cut into squares.

3.Place gently in an even layer on prepped cookie sheet. Cook for 10 minutes.

4.Cook in batches.

Nutrition: Calories: 205; Fat: 19.3g; Carbs: 2.9g; Protein: 5.3g

Crispy Keto Pork Bites

Prep Time: 20 Min | **Cook Time:** 30 Min | **Serve:** 3

- ½ pork belly, sliced to thin strips
- 1 tablespoon butter
- 1 onion, diced
- 4 tablespoons coconut cream Salt and pepper to taste

1. Place all ingredients in a mixing bowl and allow to marinate in the fridge for 2 hours.
2. When 2 hours is nearly up, preheat oven to 400oF and lightly grease a cookie sheet with cooking spray.
3. Place the pork strips in an even layer on the cookie sheet. Roast for 30 minutes and turnover halfway through cooking.

Nutrition: Calories: 448; Fat: 40.6g; Carbs: 1.9g;

Protein: 19.1g

Fat Burger Bombs

Prep Time: 30 Min | **Cook Time:** 20 Min | **Serve:** 6

- 12 slices uncured bacon, chopped
- 1 cup almond flour
- 2 eggs, beaten
- ½ pound ground beef Salt and pepper to taste 3 tablespoons olive oil

1. In a mixing bowl, combine all ingredients except for the olive oil.

2. Use your hands to form small balls with the mixture. Place in a baking sheet and allow to set in the fridge for at least 2 hours.

3. Once 2 hours is nearly up, preheat oven to 400oF.

4.Place meatballs in a single layer in a baking sheet and brush the meat balls with olive oil on all sides.

5.Cook for 20 minutes.

Nutrition: Calories: 448; Fat: 40.6g; Carbs: 1.9g; Protein: 19.1g

Onion Cheese Muffins

Prep Time: 20 Min | **Cook Time:** 20 Min | **Serve:** 6

- ¼ cup Colby jack cheese, shredded
- ¼ cup shallots, minced
- 1 cup almond flour
- 1 egg
- 3 tbsp sour cream
- ½ tsp salt
- 3 tbsp melted butter or oil

1. Line 6 muffin tins with 6 muffin liners. Set aside and preheat oven to 350oF.

2. In a bowl, stir the dry and wet ingredients alternately. Mix well using a spatula until the consistency of the mixture becomes even.

3.Scoop a spoonful of the batter to the prepared muffin tins.

Bake for 20 minutes in oven until golden brown.

Nutrition: Calories: 193; Fat: 17.4g; Carbs: 4.6g; Protein: 6.3g

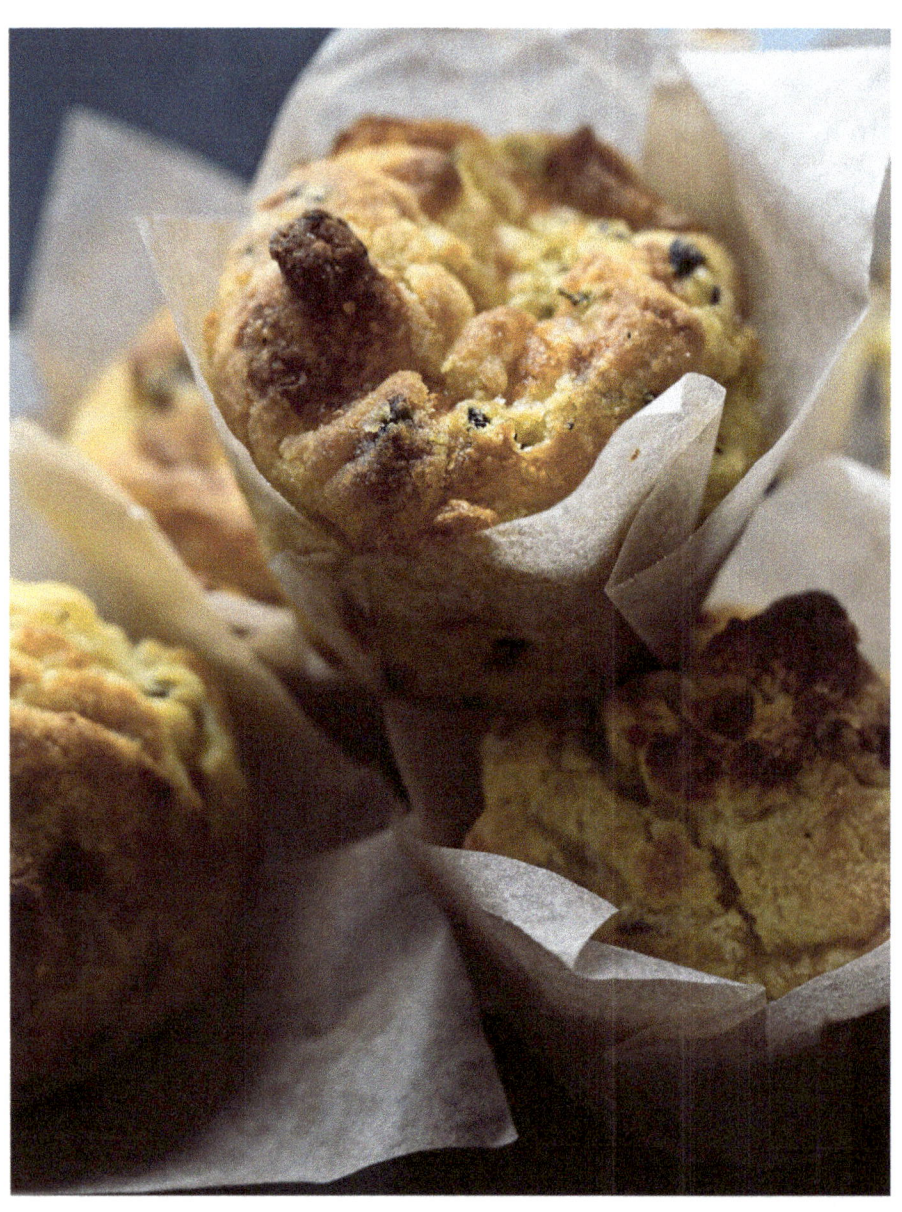

Bacon-Flavored Kale Chips

Prep Time: 20 Min | **Cook Time:** 25 Min | **Serve:** 6

- 2 tbsp butter
- ¼ cup bacon grease
- 1-lb kale, around 1 bunch
- 1 to 2 tsp salt

1. Remove the rib from kale leaves and tear into 2-inch pieces.

2. Clean the kale leaves thoroughly and dry them inside a salad spinner.

3. In a skillet, add the butter to the bacon grease and warm the two fats under low heat. Add salt and stir constantly.

4. Set aside and let it cool.

5. Put the dried kale in a Ziploc back and add the cool liquid bacon grease and butter mixture.

6. Seal the Ziploc back and gently shake the kale leaves with the butter mixture. The leaves should have this shiny consistency which means that they are coated evenly with the fat.

7. Pour the kale leaves on a cookie sheet and sprinkle more salt if necessary.

8. Bake for 25 minutes inside a preheated 350-degree oven or until the leaves start to turn brown as well as crispy.

Nutrition: Calories: 148; Fat: 13.1g; Carbs: 6.6g; Protein: 3.3g

Keto-Approved Trail Mix

Prep Time: 10 Min | **Cook Time:** 3 Min | **Serve:** 8

- ½ cup salted pumpkin seeds
- ½ cup slivered almonds
- ¾ cup roasted pecan halves
- ¾ cup unsweetened cranberries
- 1 cup toasted coconut flakes None

1.In a skillet, place almonds and pecans. Heat for 2-3 minutes and let cool. Once cooled, in a large re-sealable plastic bag, combine all ingredients. Seal and shake vigorously to mix.

Nutrition: Calories: 184; Fat: 14.4g; Carbs: 13.0g; Protein: 4.4g

Reese Cups

Prep Time: 15 Min | **Cook Time:** 1 Min | **Serve:** 12

- ½ cup unsweetened shredded coconut
- 1 cup almond butter
- 1 cup dark chocolate chips
- 1 tablespoon Stevia
- 1 tablespoon coconut oil

1. Line 12 muffin tins with 12 muffin liners.

2. Place the almond butter, honey and oil in a glass bowl and microwave for 30 seconds or until melted. Divide the mixture into 12 muffin tins. Let it cool for 30 minutes in the fridge.

3. Add the shredded coconuts and mix until evenly distributed.

4.Pour the remaining melted chocolate on top of the coconuts. Freeze for an hour.

5.Carefully remove the chocolates from the muffin tins to create perfect Reese cups.

Nutrition: Calories: 214; Fat: 17.1g; Carbs: 13.7g; Protein: 5.0g

Curry 'n Poppy Devilled Eggs

Prep Time: 20 Min | **Cook Time:** 8 Min | **Serve:** 6

- ½ cup mayonnaise
- ½ tbsp poppy seeds
- 1 tbsp red curry paste
- 6 eggs ¼ tsp salt

1. Place eggs in a small pot and add enough water to cover it. Bring to a boil without a cover, lower fire to a simmer and simmer for 8 minutes.
2. Immediately dunk in ice cold water once done cooking. Peel eggshells and slice eggs in half lengthwise.
3. Remove yolks and place them in a medium bowl. Add the rest of the ingredients in the bowl except for the egg whites. Mix well.

4.Evenly return the yolk mixture into the middle of the egg whites.

Nutrition: Calories: 200; Fat: 19.0g; Carbs: 1.0g; Protein: 6.0g

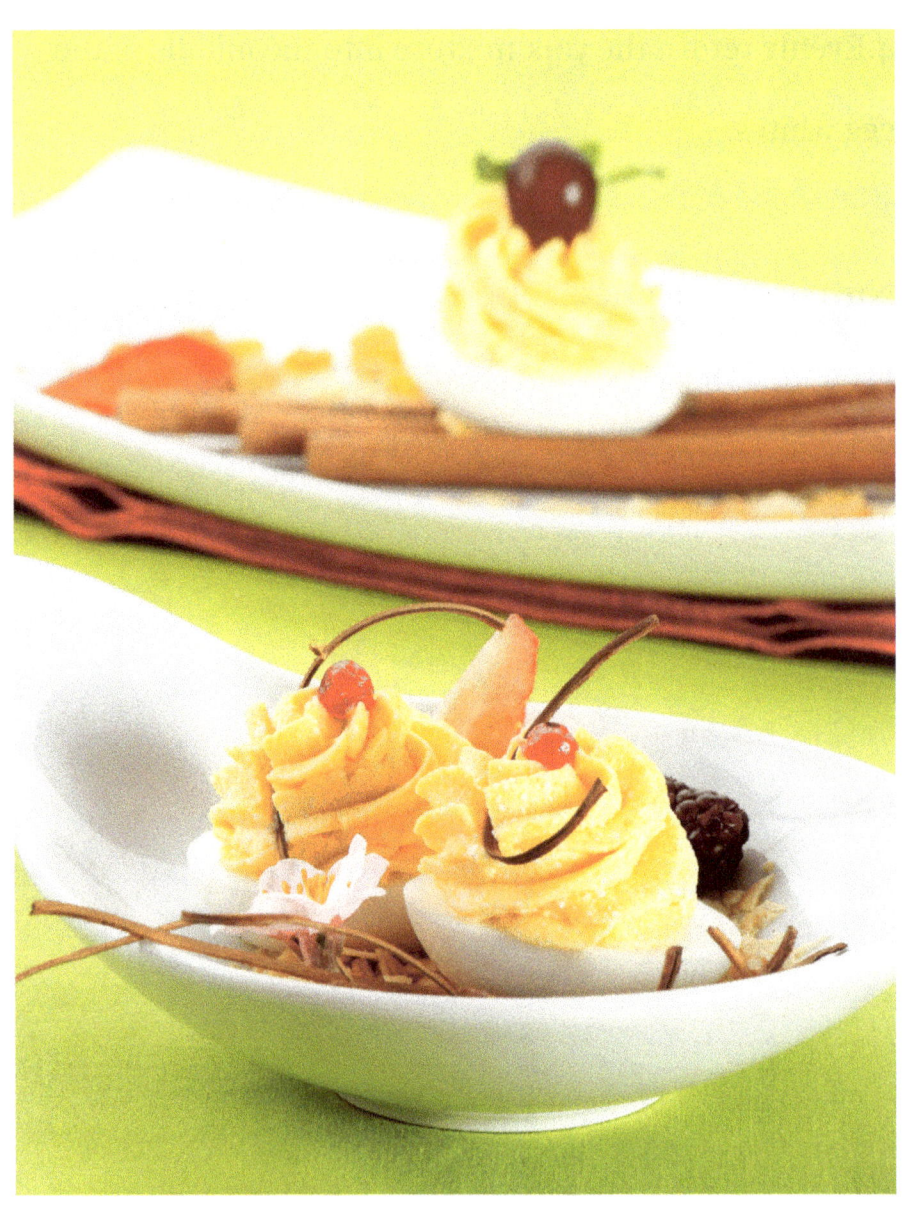

Bacon and Cheddar Cheese Balls

Prep Time: 10 Min | **Cook Time:** 8 Min | **Serve:** 10

- ½ tsp chili flakes (optional
- 5 1/3-oz bacon
- 5 1/3-oz cheddar cheese
- 5 1/3-oz cream cheese
- ½ tsp pepper

1. Pan fry bacon until crisped, around 8 minutes.

2. Meanwhile, in a food processor, process remaining ingredients. Then transfer to a bowl and refrigerate. When ready to handle, form into 20 equal balls.

3. Once bacon is cooked, crumble bacon and spread on a plate.

4.Roll the balls on the crumbled bacon to coat.

Nutrition: Calories: 225.6; Fat: 21.6g; Carbs: 1.6g; Protein: 6.4g

Cheese Roll-Ups the Keto Way

Prep Time: 15 Min | **Cook Time:** 0 Min | **Serve:** 4

- 4 slices cheddar cheese
- 4 ham slices
- None

1. Place one cheese slice on a flat surface and top with one slice of ham.

2. Roll from one end to the other. Repeat process to remaining cheese and ham.

Nutrition: Calories: 60; Fat: 2.6g; Carbs: 2.5g; Protein: 6.7g

Cheddar Cheese Chips

Prep Time: Min | **Cook Time:** 8 Min | **Serve:** 4

- 8 oz. cheddar cheese or provolone cheese or edam cheese, in slices
- ½ tsp paprika powder None

1. Line baking sheet with foil and preheat oven to 400oF.
2. Place cheese slices on baking sheet and sprinkle paprika powder on top. Pop in the oven and bake for 8 to 10 minutes.
3. Pay particular attention when timer reaches 6 to 7 minutes as a burnt cheese tastes bitter.

Nutrition: Calories: 228; Fat: 19.0g; Carbs: 2.0g; Protein: 13.0g

Cardamom and Cinnamon Fat Bombs

Prep Time: Min | **Cook Time:** 3 Min | **Serve:** 10

- ¼ tsp ground cardamom (green
- ¼ tsp ground cinnamon
- ½ cup unsweetened shredded coconut
- ½ tsp vanilla extract
- 3-oz unsalted butter, room temperature None

1. Place a nonstick pan on medium fire and toast coconut until lightly browned.
2. In a bowl, mix all ingredients.
3. Evenly roll into 10 equal balls.
4. Let it cool in the fridge.

Nutrition: Calories: 90; Fat: 10.0g; Carbs: 0.4g; Protein: 0.4g

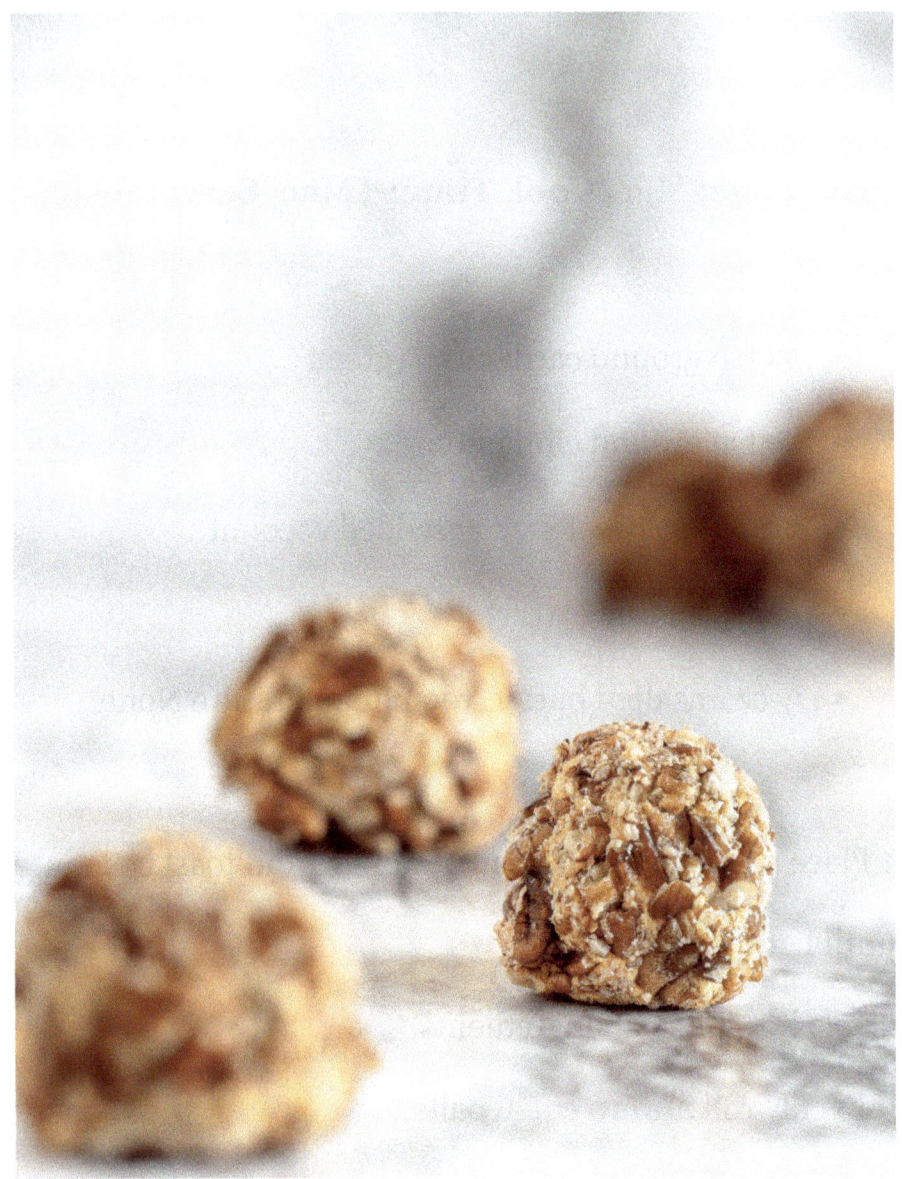

No Cook Coconut and Chocolate Bars

Prep Time: 15 Min | **Cook Time:** 0 Min | **Serve:** 6

- 1 tbsp Stevia
- ¾ cup shredded coconut, unsweetened
- ½ cup ground nuts (almonds, pecans, or walnuts
  ¼ cup unsweetened cocoa powder
- 4 tbsp coconut oil Done

1. In a medium bowl, mix shredded coconut, nuts and cocoa powder. Add Stevia and coconut oil.
2. Mix batter thoroughly.
3. In a 9x9 square inch pan or dish, press the batter and for 30-minutes place in the freezer.

Nutrition: Calories: 148; Fat: 7.8g; Carbs: 2.3g; Protein: 1.6g

Coleslaw

Prep Time: 10 minutes | **Serve:** 2

- 1 cup white cabbage
- 1 tablespoon mayonnaise
- ½ teaspoon ground black pepper
- ½ teaspoon salt

1. Shred the white cabbage and place it in the big salad bowl.

2. Sprinkle it with ground black pepper and salt.

3. Add mayonnaise and mix up coleslaw very carefully.

Nutrition: calories 39, fat 2.5, fiber 1, carbs 4.1, protein 0.6

Roasted Zucchini and Pumpkin Cubes

Prep Time: 10 min | **Cook Time:** 20 min | **Serve:** 3

- 1 cup zucchini, chopped
- ¼ cup pumpkin, chopped
- ¼ teaspoon thyme
- ½ teaspoon ground coriander
- ½ teaspoon ground cloves
- 1 tablespoon olive oil
- ½ teaspoon butter
- 1 teaspoon dried dill

1. Toss butter in the skillet and melt it.
2. Add olive oil, zucchini, and pumpkin.

3.Start to roast vegetables over the medium heat for 5 minutes.

4.Hen sprinkle them with thyme, ground coriander, ground cloves, and dried dill.

5.Mix up well and close the lid.

6.Cook the vegetables on the low heat for 15 minutes.

Nutrition: calories 66, fat 5.5, fiber 1.2, carbs 3.4, protein 0.8

Chile Casserole

Prep Time: 15 min | **Cook Time:** 15 min | **Serve:** 4

- 1 cup chili peppers, green, raw
- 1 teaspoon olive oil
- 3 oz Cheddar cheese, shredded
- 1 teaspoon butter
- 2 eggs, whisked
- ¼ cup heavy cream ½ teaspoon salt

1. Preheat the grill well and place chili peppers on it.

2. Grill the chili peppers for 5 minutes. Stir them from time to time. Then chill the peppers little and peel them. Remove the seeds. Place the peppers in the casserole tray.

3.Add butter and sprinkle with salt.

4.In the separated bowl, mix up together heavy cream, whisked eggs, and cheese.

5.Pour the liquid over the chili peppers and transfer casserole in the [reheated to the 365F oven.

6.Cook casserole for 10 minutes.

Nutrition: calories 169, fat 14.2, fiber 0.3, carbs 2.4, protein 8.6

Pickled Jalapeno

Prep Time: 10 min | **Cook Time:** 10 min | **Serve:** 6

- 6 jalapeno peppers

- ¼ cup apple cider vinegar 1/3 cup water

- ¼ teaspoon peppercorns

- 1 garlic clove, peeled

- ½ teaspoon ground coriander

1. Pour apple cider vinegar in the saucepan.

2. Add water, peppercorns, and bring the liquid to boil. Wash the jalapeno peppers and slice them.

3. Put the sliced jalapenos in the glass jar. Add ground cinnamon and garlic clove.

4.After this, add boiled apple cider vinegar liquid and close the lid. Marinate the jalapenos as a minimum for 1 hour.

Nutrition: calories 9, fat 0.2, fiber 0.6, carbs 1.4, protein 0.2

Naan

Prep Time: 10 min | **Cook Time:** 4 min | **Serve:** 2

- 1 tablespoon butter
- 1 tablespoon almond flour
- ¾ teaspoon baking powder ¼ teaspoon lemon juice
- 1 teaspoon coconut oil, softened
- 1 teaspoon psyllium husk powder

1. In the mixing bowl, mix up almond flour, baking powder, lemon juice, coconut oil, and psyllium husk powder.
2. Knead the dough and cut it into 2 pieces.
3. Roll up the dough pieces to get naan bread shape.
4. Toss butter in the skillet and bring it to boil.

5.Place naan bread in the preheated butter and roast for 1 minute from each side.

6.The time of cooking depends on the naan size.

Nutrition: calories 157, fat 15.1, fiber 2.7, carbs 5.2, protein 3.1

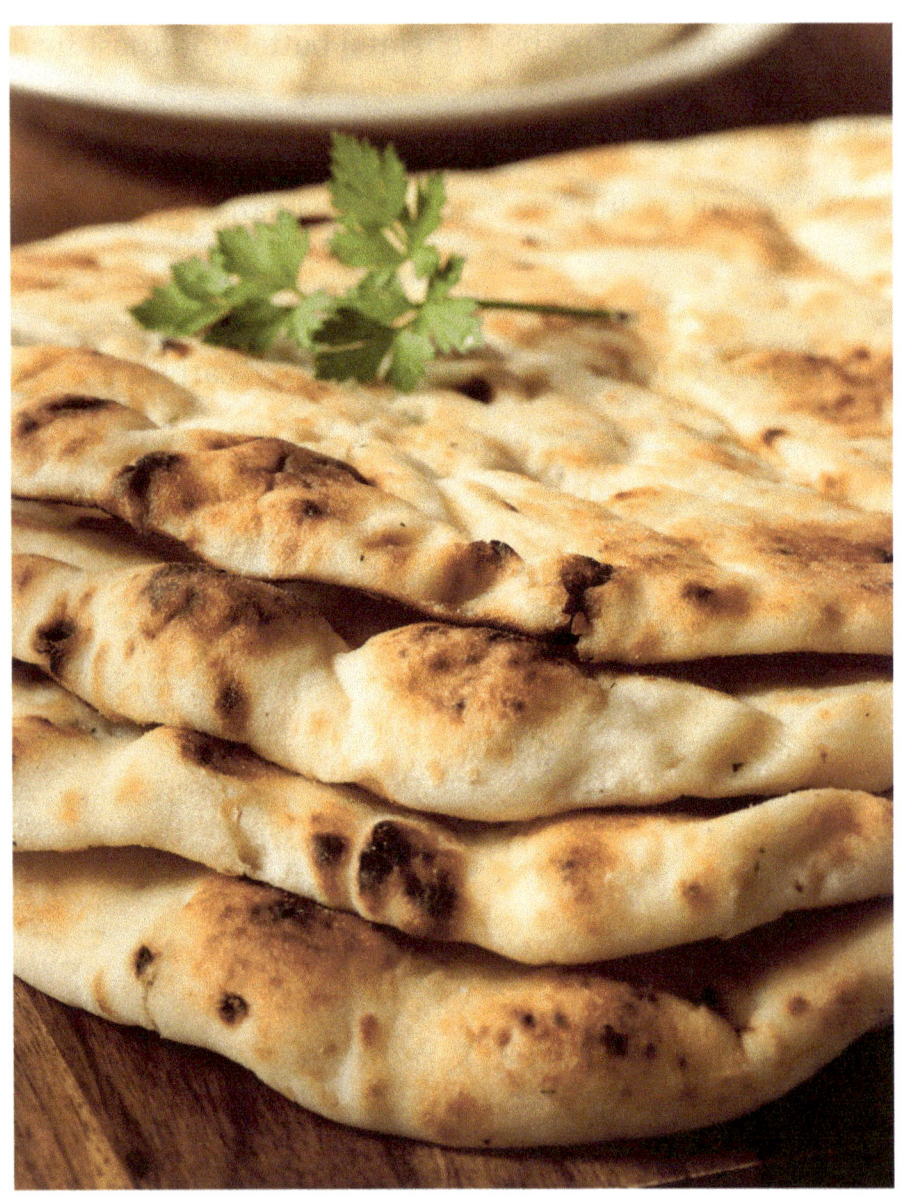

Sauteed Tomato Cabbage

Prep Time: 10 min | **Cook Time:** 35 min | **Serve:** 4

- 1 tablespoon tomato paste
- 1 bell pepper, chopped
- ½ oz celery, grated
- 2 cups white cabbage, shredded
- 1 tablespoon butter
- 1 tablespoon dried oregano
- 1/3 cup water
- ¼ cup coconut cream
- 1 teaspoon salt

1.Mix up together tomato paste, coconut cream, and water. Pour the liquid in the saucepan.

2.Add bell pepper, grated celery, white cabbage, butter, and dried oregano. Sprinkle the mixture with salt and mix up gently.

3.Close the lid and saute cabbage for 35 minutes over the medium-low heat.

Nutrition: calories 86, fat 6.7, fiber 2.3, carbs 6.7, protein 1.4

Tender Radicchio

Prep Time: 10 min | **Cook Time:** 8 min | **Serve:** 4

- 8 oz radicchio
- 1 teaspoon canola oil
- ½ teaspoon apple cider vinegar ¼ cup heavy cream
- 1 teaspoon minced garlic
- 1 teaspoon dried dill

1.Slice the radicchio into 4 slices.

2.Line the baking dish with parchment and put sliced radicchio on it. Sprinkle the vegetables with canola oil, apple cider vinegar, and dried dill. Bake radicchio in the preheated to the 360F oven for 8 minutes. Meanwhile, whisk together heavy cream with minced garlic.

3.Transfer the cooked radicchio on the plates and sprinkle with minced heavy cream mixture.

Nutrition: calories 43, fat 4, fiber 0.2, carbs 1.5, protein 0.5

Green Salad with Walnuts

Prep Time: 10 min | **Serve:** 2

- 1 cup arugula
- 2 tablespoons walnuts, chopped
- 1 tablespoon avocado oil
- ½ teaspoon sesame seeds
- 1 teaspoon lemon juice
- ½ teaspoon lemon zest, grated
- 1 tomato, chopped

1.Chop arugula roughly and put in the salad bowl. Add walnuts, sesame seeds, and chopped tomato.

2.Make the dressing: mix up together avocado oil, sesame seeds, lemon juice, and grated lemon zest.

3.Pour the dressing over salad and shake it gently.

Nutrition: calories 71, fat 6, fiber 1.5, carbs 3.1, protein 2.7

Jicama Slaw

Prep Time: 10 minutes | **Serve:** 4

- 1 cup jicama, julienned
- 1 bell pepper, julienned
- 1 onion, sliced
- 1 tablespoon fresh cilantro, chopped
- ½ carrot, julienned
- 2 tablespoons olive oil
- 1 teaspoon apple cider vinegar
- ½ teaspoon cayenne pepper
- ½ teaspoon salt
- 1/3 cup red cabbage, shredded
- ¼ teaspoon liquid stevia Directions:

1. In the mixing bowl, combine jicama, bell pepper, sliced onion, fresh cilantro, carrot, olive oil, apple cider vinegar, and liquid stevia. Mix up the salad mixture.

2. Then sprinkle slaw with cayenne pepper, salt, and red cabbage.

3. Mix up the cooked slaw one more time and transfer on the plates.

Nutrition: calories 98, fat 7.2, fiber 2.9, carbs 8.7, protein 1

Peanut Slaw

Prep Time: 10 min | **Serve:** 4

- 1 cup white cabbage
- 1 teaspoon peanut butter
- 1 teaspoon lemon juice
- 1 tablespoon peanuts, chopped
- ½ teaspoon ground black pepper
- 1 tablespoon canola oil
- 1 oz scallions, chopped
- 1 teaspoon sriracha
- ¼ cup fresh parsley, chopped

1. Shred the white cabbage and transfer in the mixing bowl. Add peanuts, chopped fresh parsley, and scallions.

2.Then make the slaw dressing: whisk together peanut butter, lemon juice, ground black pepper, and canola oil.

3.Pour the dressing over the white cabbage mixture.

4.Add sriracha and chopped parsley.

5.Shake the slaw gently and transfer on the plates.

Nutrition: calories 62, fat 5.4, fiber 1.1, carbs 2.9, protein 1.4

White Mushroom Saute

Prep Time: 15 min | **Cook Time:** 25 min | **Serve:** 6

- 10 oz white mushrooms, chopped
- 1 carrot, chopped
- 1 onion, chopped
- ½ cup of water
- 3 tablespoons coconut cream
- 1 teaspoon salt
- ½ teaspoon turmeric
- 1 teaspoon chili flakes
- 1 teaspoon coconut oil
- ½ teaspoon Italian seasoning

1. In the saucepan, combine white mushrooms, chopped carrot, onion, and mix up gently.

2. Sprinkle the vegetables with coconut cream, salt, turmeric, chili flakes, and coconut oil.

3. Add Italian seasoning and mix up well.

4. Cook the mixture over the high heat for 5 minutes.

5. Stir the vegetables constantly.

6. Then add water and close the lid.

7. Saute the meal for 20 minutes over the medium heat.

8. Then let saute rest for 10 minutes before.

Nutrition: calories 47, fat 2.9, fiber 1.3, carbs 4.9, protein 1.9

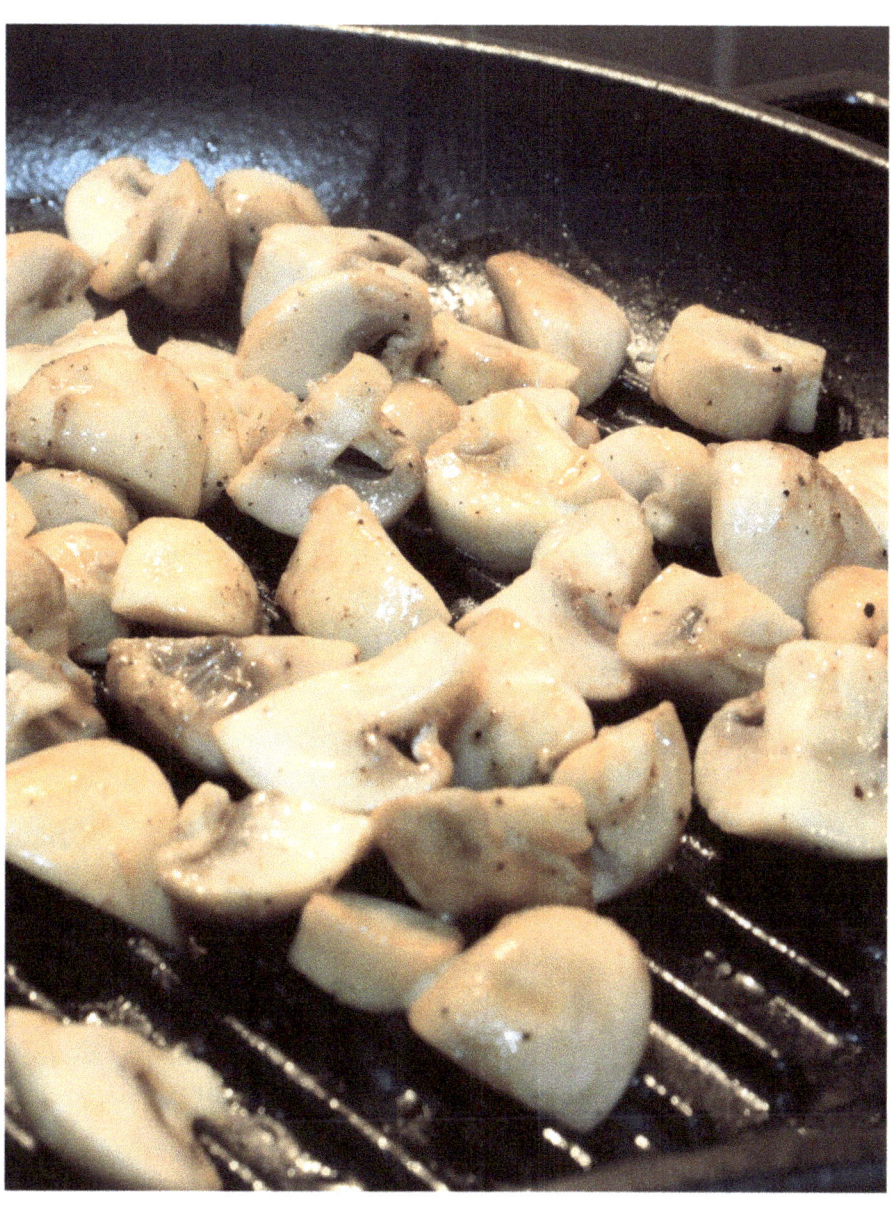

Caesar Salad

Prep Time: 15 minutes | **Serve:** 5

- 1 tablespoon capers
- 2 cups lettuce, chopped
- 1 teaspoon walnuts, chopped
- 1 teaspoon mustard
- 2 tablespoons canola oil
- 1 teaspoon lime juice
- ½ teaspoon white pepper
- 1 avocado, peeled, chopped

1. Place walnuts, mustard, canola oil, lime juice, white pepper, and avocado in the blender.
2. Blend the mixture until smooth.

3.After this, transfer the avocado smooth mixture in the salad bowl.

4.Add chopped lettuce.

5.Sprinkle the salad with capers. Don't stir the salad before.

Nutrition: calories 142, fat 14, fiber 3.1, carbs 4.6, protein 1.2

Cranberry Relish

Prep Time: 5 min | **Serve:** 6

- 1 cup cranberries
- 1 orange, peeled, chopped
- 1 tablespoon Erythritol
- 3 tablespoons lemon juice

1. Place cranberries and chopped orange in the blender.
2. Add Erythritol and lemon juice.
3. Pulse the ingredients for 1 minute.
4. Transfer the relish in the plate.
5. The side dish tastes the best with meat meals.

Nutrition: calories 26, fat 0.1, fiber 1.4 carbs 5.4, protein 0.4

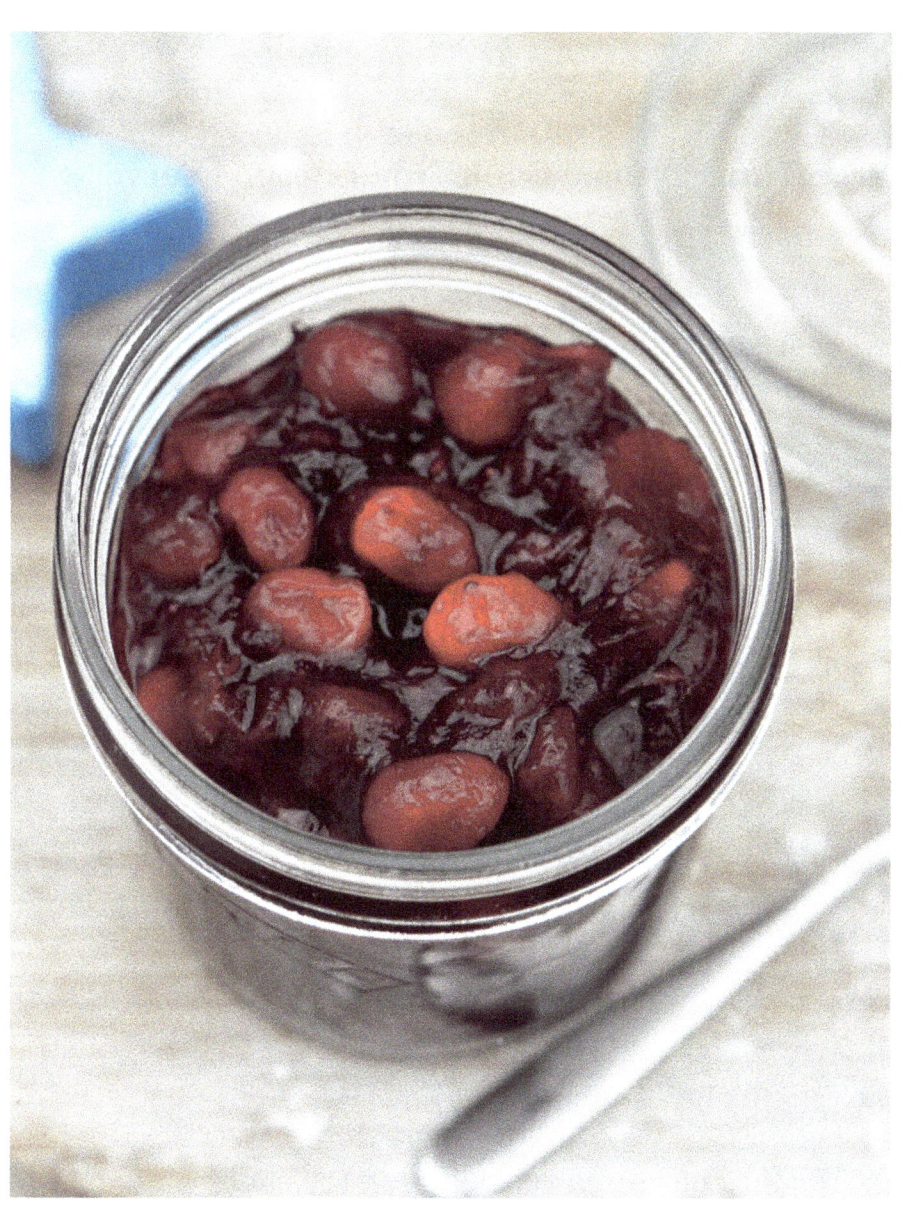

Vegetable Tots

Prep Time: 15 min | **Cook Time:** 12 min | **Serve:** 8

- 2 cups cauliflower
- 1 cup broccoli
- 4 eggs
- 1/3 cup almond flour
- 3 oz Parmesan, grated
- 1 teaspoon ground coriander
- ½ teaspoon ground thyme
- 1 teaspoon olive oil

1.Grate the broccoli and cauliflower.

2.Transfer the grated vegetables in the cheesecloth and squeeze the liquid. Then put vegetables in the mixing bowl.

3. Beat the eggs in the mixture and add grated cheese.

4. Then add almond flour, ground coriander, ground thyme, and mix it up.

5. Line the baking tray with baking paper and brush with 1 teaspoon of olive oil.

6. Make the medium size tots from the vegetable mixture and put them in the baking tray.

7. Bake the vegetable tots for 12 minutes at 365F.

8. Chill the meal to the room temperature before.

Nutrition: calories 88, fat 5.7, fiber 1.1, carbs 2.9, protein 7.3

Hasselback Zucchini

Prep Time: 15 min | **Cook Time:** 20 min | **Serve:** 3

- 3 small zucchini
- 4 oz Parmesan, sliced
- 1 tablespoon cream
- ½ teaspoon chili flakes
- ½ teaspoon butter
- ½ teaspoon ground black pepper
- ½ teaspoon olive oil

1. Trim zucchini and cut them in the shape of the Hasselback.

2. Fill the zucchini Hasselback with sliced Parmesan.

3. Then whisk together cream, chili flakes, butter, ground

black pepper, and olive oil.

4.Brush the zucchini with the cream mixture generously.

5.Wrap the zucchini Hasselback in the foil.

6.Preheat the oven to 365F.

7.Put the wrapped zucchini in the oven and cook for 20 minutes.

8.When the time is over, chill the zucchini for 5 minutes and then discard the foil.

9.Transfer the meal on the plates.

Nutrition: calories 156, fat 9.9, fiber 1.4, carbs 5.7, protein 13.7

Lime Fennel Bulb

Prep Time: 10 min | **Cook Time:** 15 min | **Serve:** 4

- 9 oz fennel bulb
- ½ lime
- 2 tablespoons butter
- 1 teaspoon olive oil
- 1 teaspoon harissa
- ½ teaspoon salt

1. Cut every fennel bulb into 4 pieces.

2. Sprinkle the fennel with olive oil, harissa, and salt. Massage the fennel pieces with the help of the fingertips and transfer in the tray.

3. Add butter and bake fennel for 15 minutes at 360F. Stir the vegetables once during cooking.

Nutrition: calories 87, fat 7.3, fiber 2.2, carbs 6, protein 1

Baked Garlic

Prep Time: 5 min | **Cook Time:** 20 min | **Serve:** 3

- 3 big garlic cloves, peeled
- 3 teaspoons olive oil
- 1 teaspoon salt
- ½ teaspoon apple cider vinegar

1.Place the garlic cloves in the parchment. Add olive oil, salt, and apple cider vinegar.

2.Wrap the garlic to get the parchment pocket and place it in the oven. Cook the garlic for 20 minutes at 355F.

3.When the time is over, the garlic should be very soft. Serve the garlic with all remaining gravy.

Nutrition: calories 54, fat 4.7, fiber 0.2, carbs 3, protein 0.6

Roasted Okra

Prep Time: 10 min | **Cook Time:** 15 min | **Serve:** 4

- 1 ½ cup okra
- 1 tablespoon almond flour
- 1 teaspoon salt
- 1 tablespoon coconut oil
- ½ teaspoon cayenne pepper
- ½ teaspoon dried cilantro
- 1 tablespoon heavy cream

1. Slice the okra roughly.

2. Put coconut oil in the skillet.

3. Add sliced okra and start to cook it over the medium-high heat. Sprinkle the vegetables with salt, cayenne

pepper, and dried cilantro. Then add heavy cream and mix up well.

4.Cook okra for 5 minutes more.

5.Sprinkle the vegetables with almond flour and close the lid.

6.Cook the side dish for 5 minutes over the medium heat.

Nutrition: calories 98, fat 8.4, fiber 2, carbs 4.5, protein 2.3

Broccoli Gratin

Prep Time: 10 min | **Cook Time:** 30 min | **Serve:** 6

- 2 cups broccoli florets
- 1 teaspoon salt
- 1 teaspoon chili flakes
- 3 eggs, whisked
- 2 oz Swiss cheese, grated
- 1 onion, diced
- 1 cup heavy cream

1.Whisk together chili flakes, salt, eggs, and heavy cream.

2.Add the diced onion in the mixture and stir gently.

3.After this, place broccoli florets into the non-sticky gratin mold.

4.Sprinkle the vegetables with Swiss cheese and heavy cream mixture.

5.Cover the gratin with foil and secure the edges.

6.Cook gratin for 30 minutes in the preheated to the 360F oven.

7.When the time is over, discard the foil and check if the broccoli is tender.

8.Chill the gratin little and transfer on the plates.

Nutrition: calories 154, fat 12.3, fiber 1.2, carbs 5, protein 6.8

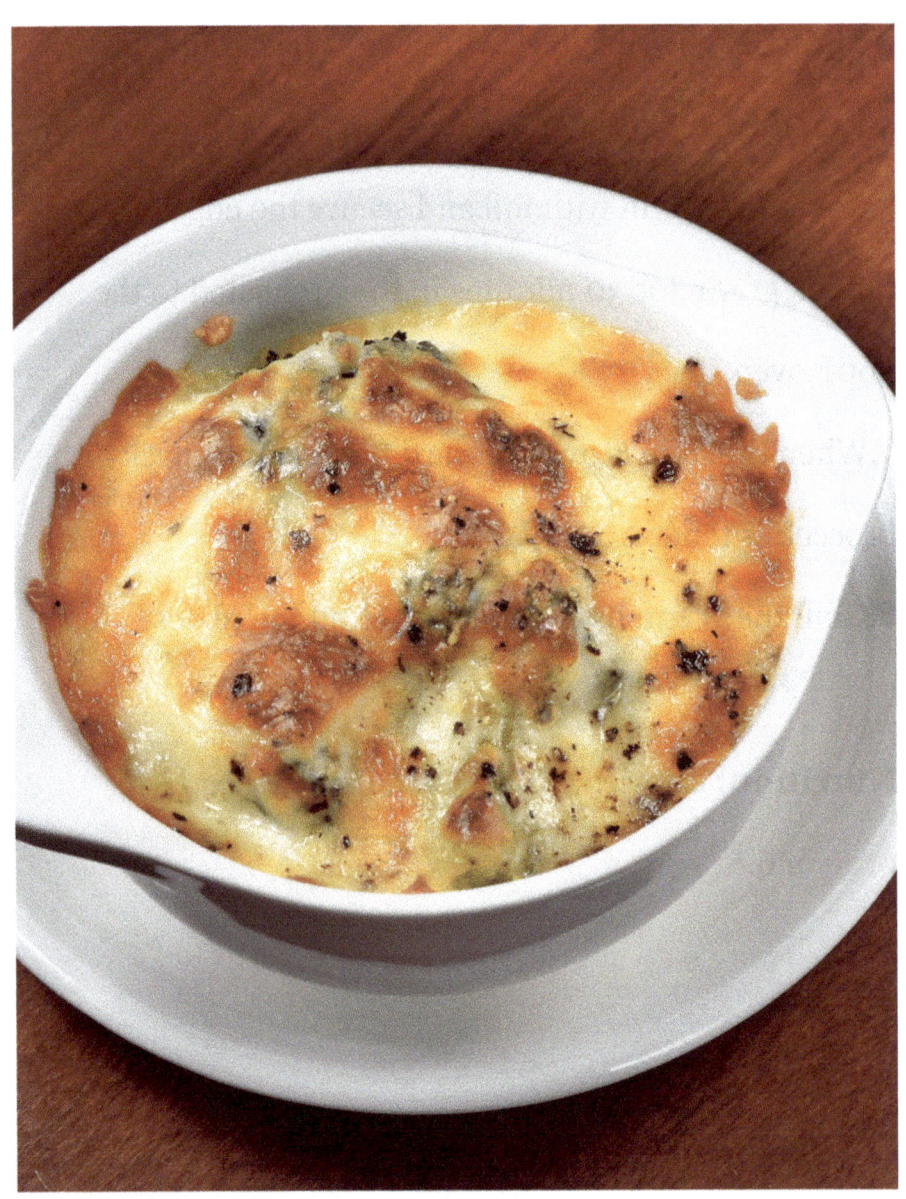

Cayenne Pepper Green Beans

Prep Time: 10 min | **Cook Time:** 20 min | **Serve:** 4

- 1 teaspoon cayenne pepper
- 1 pound green beans, trimmed and halved
- 1 tablespoon avocado oil
- 2 cups of water

1. Bring the water to boil and add green beans. Cook them for 10 minutes.

2. Then remove water and add avocado oil and cayenne pepper.

3. Roast the vegetables for 2-3 minutes on high heat.

Nutrition: 41 calories, 2.2g protein, 8.5g carbohydrates, 0.7g fat, 4.1g fiber, 0mg cholesterol, 11mg sodium, 258mg potassium.

www.ingramcontent.com/pod-product-compliance
Lightning Source LLC
Chambersburg PA
CBHW070725030426
42336CB00013B/1921